INSOMNIAC'S COMPANION

Calming Stories for Restless Adults

Nolan Marks

Foreword

Dear Reader,

Welcome to "Insomniac's Companion: Calming Stories for Restless Adults." I'm Nolan Marks, and I created this collection of soothing stories to help you relax and unwind at the end of a long day. In today's fast-paced world, sleep often seems elusive, and finding moments of tranquility can be challenging. My hope is that these stories will provide a gentle escape from daily stress and guide you towards a restful night's sleep.

Each story in this collection has been carefully crafted to be interesting enough to hold your attention, yet not too exciting to keep you awake. To get the most out of this book, I recommend the following steps:

1. Set the scene: Ensure your reading environment is conducive to relaxation by using warm, soft lighting that is still bright enough for you to read comfortably. Dimming the lights or using a bedside lamp can create a calming atmosphere.

2. Prepare yourself: Before you begin reading, take a few deep breaths, allowing yourself to release any tension in your body and mind. This simple act can help you ease into the world of the story and be more receptive to its calming effects.

3.   Immerse yourself: As you read each story, allow yourself to be fully present and let the soothing narratives envelop you.

4.   Reflect and unwind: After finishing a story, switch off the lights, close your eyes, and try to recall the images and emotions the story evoked. Let these gentle thoughts guide you into a peaceful slumber.

If you enjoy this book, I would be grateful if you considered leaving a positive review on Amazon. Your support truly means the world to a self-published author like me. By sharing your experience, you'll help others discover the calming power of these stories, too.

I wish you many nights of peaceful rest and hope these stories become a cherished companion on your journey to a better night's sleep.

Sweet dreams,

Nolan Marks

Insomniac's Companion

The Seashell Collector

As the first light of dawn kissed the horizon, Evelyn set out for her morning walk along the shoreline. The soft, golden sand was still cool beneath her feet, and the air carried the briny scent of the sea. The rhythmic sound of waves lapping against the shore accompanied her as she strolled along the water's edge, her eyes scanning the beach for treasures left behind by the retreating tide.

Evelyn had always been fascinated by seashells. Each one was a small, unique work of art, shaped by the elements and the myster ious depths of the ocean. She marveled at their intricate patterns, diverse textures, and the stories they held within their delicate forms. The beach had become her sanctuary, a place where she could escape from the hustle and bustle of everyday life and lose herself in the peaceful embrace of nature.

As she walked, she spotted a small, spiraled shell half-buried in the sand. Gently brushing away the grains, she revealed a stunning conch, its surface adorned with a kaleidoscope of colors that shimmered in the early morning light. She wondered about the creature that once called this shell home and the journey it took before finding its way to this beach. Perhaps it had traveled thousands of miles, carried by the whims of the currents, before finally coming to rest at her feet.

Evelyn continued her search, uncovering an array of seashells in various shapes and sizes. Each new discovery was a testament to the ocean's boundless creativity. With each shell, she pondered the vastness of the sea and the secrets it concealed beneath its surface. The endless ebb and flow of the tides, the unseen world of marine life, and the countless stories waiting to be uncovered all captivated her imagination.

As she wandered further down the beach, Evelyn stumbled upon a small tide pool, its calm waters sheltering a microcosm of life. Tiny fish darted among the rocks, and brightly colored sea anemones swayed gently in the current. As she knelt down for a closer look, she discovered a fragile scallop shell, its iridescent interior glistening like a precious gem. She couldn't help but smile at the delicate beauty of her find and the serendipity of this moment.

The sun climbed higher in the sky, casting a warm glow over the beach as Evelyn walked along the shoreline, her collection of shells growing with each step. The gentle sound of the waves, like a soothing lullaby, brought a sense of peace and serenity to her heart. She felt a deep connection to the ocean, its constant presence a reminder of the ever-changing nature of life.

As the morning slipped away, Evelyn found herself lost in thought. The seashells she collected seemed to hold within them the essence of the sea itself—its vastness, its power, and its tranquility. Each shell was a symbol of resilience and adaptation, a testament to the perseverance of life in the face of adversity. She felt humbled by these small tokens of nature's beauty and strength, and they served as a gentle reminder to find the extraordinary in the ordinary.

As her walk came to an end, Evelyn looked out at the horizon, where the sky met the sea in a dance of colors. She thought about the shells she had collected, each one with its own unique story and beauty. In that moment, she felt a profound connection to the ocean and its endless wonders, grateful for the simple pleasure of combing the beach for these small, yet precious treasures.

With a contented smile, Evelyn placed the shells carefully in her woven bag and turned to leave, knowing that tomorrow would bring new discoveries and more stories to ponder, all hidden within the fragile beauty of seashells. As she made her way back home, the sun's warmth on her skin and the gentle sea breeze rustling through her hair, she felt a deep sense of gratitude for these tranquil moments spent in the embrace of the ocean.

Over the coming weeks and months, Evelyn continued her morning ritual of walking the beach, each day uncovering new treasures and marveling at the ocean's endless gifts. Her collection grew, filling her home with the comforting presence of the sea. She arranged her finds in delicate displays, creating a tangible reminder of the peace and serenity she found during her beachcombing adventures.

As the seasons changed, so too did the beach. Summer's warmth gave way to autumn's vibrant colors, and the once-busy shoreline grew quiet and still. Yet, even in the cool embrace of fall, Evelyn found solace in the ever-present rhythm of the waves and the enduring beauty of the seashells.

Winter arrived, cloaking the beach in a blanket of frost and transforming the landscape into a world of crystalline beauty. The cold air stung her cheeks as she walked, but she found warmth in the knowledge that the ocean's treasures still lay hidden beneath the sand, waiting to be discovered when the world thawed once more.

As spring returned, bringing with it new life and the promise of renewal, Evelyn felt a profound connection to the cycle of nature, the ebb and flow of time echoing the rhythms of the ocean. The shells she collected served as a testament to this eternal dance, their fragile beauty a constant reminder of the wonder and magic that existed in the world, if only one took the time to look.

With each new day, Evelyn continued her morning walks, always seeking, always discovering. And as she wandered the shoreline, her heart filled with the gentle music of the waves and the quiet whispers of the seashells, she knew she had found a place where she could truly find peace and solace—a sanctuary by the sea.

The Quiet Café

As the first light of morning filtered through the narrow streets, casting long shadows on the cobblestones, Thomas made his way to the small, local café that had become his refuge from the world. The familiar chime of the doorbell announced his arrival, and the comforting scent of freshly brewed coffee and baked pastries enveloped him as he stepped inside.

The café was a cozy, intimate space, filled with the soft hum of conversation and the gentle clink of porcelain cups against saucers. Thomas felt a sense of familiarity and warmth in the worn wooden floors, the mismatched chairs, and the well-loved bookshelves that lined the walls. Every detail of the café seemed to have a story of its own, from the faded wallpaper adorned with intricate floral patterns to the vintage photographs and paintings that graced the walls, each one a silent witness to the countless moments that had unfolded within these walls.

As Thomas took in the sights and sounds of the café, he noticed the small, loving touches that made the space so inviting: the fresh flowers arranged in simple glass vases on each table, the soft glow of the antique lamps casting a warm, amber light, and the carefully curated selection of books and magazines that beckoned patrons to linger and lose themselves in their pages. The atmosphere was one of timeless charm and quiet contemplation, a place where the hurried pace of the outside world seemed to slow and grow still.

Thomas found his favorite spot in the corner, a small table tucked away from the bustle, where he could watch the world go by through the large windows that framed the street. The morning sunlight streamed in, casting a golden glow over the room and warming his face as he settled into the worn leather chair. With a contented sigh, he turned his attention to the menu, a simple yet elegant list of beverages and pastries that changed with the seasons and the whims of the talented barista.

As he sipped his rich, steaming coffee, Thomas allowed the familiar sounds of the café to wash over him. He found solace in the soft murmur of conversations, the gentle clatter of dishes, and the soothing notes of the jazz music playing in the background. Each sound was a thread in the tapestry of life, a reminder of the connections and shared experiences that bound them all together.

With each visit to the café, Thomas found himself drawn to the stories that unfolded around him. The elderly couple who sat by the window, sharing a pot of tea and reminiscing about their years together; the young writer, furiously scribbling in her notebook as she chased the tail of an elusive idea; the mother and daughter who shared a slice of cake and whispered secrets over steaming cups of hot chocolate—all of them found a home within these walls, each with their own unique narrative to share.

As the morning progressed, Thomas took the time to truly immerse himself in the sensory experience of the café. He inhaled the rich, earthy scent of freshly ground coffee beans, the sweet aroma of cinnamon and vanilla wafting from the glass display case filled with an assortment of pastries. He listened to the gentle hiss of the espresso machine and the melodic chime of the doorbell as new patrons arrived, each one adding their own unique voice to the symphony of sounds that filled the room.

Thomas often brought a book or a newspaper to read, but he found that the real stories were happening all around him, in the laughter and the tears, the quiet moments of reflection, and the animated conversations that filled the air. The café was a microcosm of the world outside, a place where people from all walks of life could come together and find solace in the simple act of sharing a warm beverage and a moment of connection.

As he continued to observe and savor the atmosphere, Thomas paid attention to the myriad textures that surrounded him: the smooth, cool surface of the marble countertop; the rough grain of the wooden tabletop, worn smooth by years of use; the plush velvet of the cushioned chairs, inviting patrons to sink into their embrace. He even noticed the intricate patterns of the lace curtains that filtered the sunlight, casting dappled shadows on the walls and floors. Each detail served as a reminder of the care and love that had been poured into this little corner of the world.

The passage of time seemed to slow as Thomas immersed himself in the sensory experience of the café. He lingered over his coffee, taking small sips and savoring the robust flavors and the velvety texture on his tongue. He treated himself to a buttery croissant, delighting in the delicate layers of pastry that seemed to melt in his mouth. And as the sun rose higher in the sky, the golden light of morning gradually gave way to the soft, diffuse glow of afternoon.

As the day unfolded, Thomas found himself lost in thought, his mind wandering through memories and dreams as the world outside the café continued its frenetic pace. He watched as the patrons came and went, each one leaving behind a trace of their presence in the form of an empty cup or a crumpled napkin. He realized that, in many ways, the café was a reflection of life itself: a constant ebb and flow of people, stories, and emotions, all brought together by the simple pleasures of a warm beverage and a moment of shared connection.

As the afternoon shadows grew longer, Thomas savored the last drops of his coffee, the robust flavors lingering on his tongue as he gazed out the window at the world beyond. He thought about the stories he had witnessed and the connections he had made within these walls, and he felt a profound sense of gratitude for the quiet haven that the café provided.

With a reluctant sigh, Thomas rose from his seat and gathered his belongings, preparing to rejoin the bustling world outside. But as he stepped out onto the cobblestone street, the café's comforting aroma still clinging to his clothes, he knew that this little sanctuary would always be waiting for him—a place of warmth, solace, and the simple joy of a perfectly brewed cup of coffee. And with each return to this haven of peace, he would continue to find new stories, new connections, and new moments of quiet contemplation amidst the ever-changing tapestry of life.

The Gentle Gardener

Edward stepped out into the gentle morning light, the dew still clinging to the vibrant green blades of grass beneath his feet. It was in these quiet moments, just as the world was beginning to awaken, that he found solace in his peaceful garden, a sanctuary he had lovingly tended to for many years. Since his retirement, the garden had become both a refuge from the world and a testament to the beauty of nature's delicate balance.

As he surveyed his little kingdom, Edward marveled at the myriad colors and textures that greeted him: the velvety petals of the roses, the delicate tendrils of the climbing vines, and the sturdy, rough bark of the ancient oak tree that stood sentinel over it all. Each plant had its own story to tell, and he had come to know them all intimately, nurturing them from tiny seeds or fragile cuttings into the thriving, beautiful specimens they had become.

With a sense of reverence, Edward began his morning ritual, the gentle rhythm of gardening tasks that had become as familiar and comforting as a well-worn pair of gloves. He moved gracefully from one bed to another, his hands deftly tending to the needs of each plant: watering, pruning, weeding, and feeding. Each task was performed with care and precision, a silent communion between gardener and garden that spoke of a deep, abiding love for the natural world.

As the days and weeks slipped by, Edward took quiet pleasure in observing the subtle changes that unfolded within his garden. The first tender buds of spring gave way to the riotous blooms of summer, a symphony of color and fragrance that filled the air with the sweet perfume of jasmine, lavender, and roses. The bees and butterflies danced from flower to flower, their delicate wings shimmering in the sunlight as they carried out their vital work, and Edward felt a profound sense of wonder at the intricate web of life that thrived within his little corner of the world.

As the seasons changed, so too did the garden, each new phase bringing its own unique beauty and charm. The autumn months heralded a transformation, as the once-vibrant greens turned to rich shades of gold and crimson, the leaves of the trees and shrubs painting the landscape in a breathtaking display of nature's artistry. Edward took the time to savor these moments, to appreciate the fleeting beauty of the falling leaves and the gentle sigh of the wind as it whispered through the branches.

Winter brought its own stark beauty, as the garden lay dormant beneath a blanket of frost and snow. The once-busy landscape grew still and silent, a world of icy crystal and frozen earth that seemed to hold its breath, waiting for the return of warmth and life. In these cold, quiet months, Edward found solace in the knowledge that beneath the frozen surface, the roots of his beloved plants were resting and gathering strength, preparing for the rebirth of spring and the return of the garden's vibrant tapestry.

As the cycle of the seasons continued, Edward found a deep sense of connection to the natural world, the gentle rhythm of his gardening tasks echoing the timeless dance of growth, decay, and renewal. He marveled at the intricate balance of life that existed within his garden, from the smallest insect to the mightiest tree, each one playing its part in the grand symphony of existence.

With each passing year, Edward's love for his garden grew, as did the sense of peace and contentment that he found within its sheltering embrace. In the quiet moments spent tending to his plants, he discovered a world of simple joys and profound beauty, a sanctuary where he could escape the clamor of the world and find solace in the gentle, nurturing embrace of nature.

And so, as the seasons turned and the garden continued to flourish and evolve, Edward too found a sense of growth and renewal within himself. The hours spent nurturing his plants, observing the delicate balance of nature, and reveling in the quiet moments of reflection had a profound impact on his soul, bringing him a sense of calm and tranquility that he had never known before.

In the garden, Edward found solace not only in the physical act of gardening but also in the deep connection to the earth and the cycle of life it provided. He began to see his own life as part of this larger tapestry, understanding that each season, each moment, held its own unique beauty and significance. This wisdom, gleaned from the soil and the plants that grew within it, allowed him to approach each day with a sense of gratitude and wonder, embracing the ever-changing landscape of his own existence with grace and acceptance.

As the years passed and the garden matured, it became a reflection of Edward's own journey, a living testament to the passage of time and the gentle persistence of life. The once-tender saplings had grown into strong, resilient trees, their branches reaching towards the sky in a silent celebration of growth and transformation. The flower beds, once filled with fragile seedlings, now bloomed with the vibrant colors and fragrances of a well-tended, thriving garden.

And as Edward walked the familiar paths of his sanctuary, his hands weathered and strong from years of dedicated care, he knew that his garden had become more than just a refuge from the world. It was a living, breathing testament to the power of nature and the simple, enduring beauty of life's ever-changing tapestry.

In the quiet moments of contemplation, as he knelt in the soft earth, tending to the needs of his beloved plants, Edward found a sense of purpose and connection that transcended the boundaries of his garden. He understood that the lessons learned within this sacred space had the power to transform not only his own life but also the world beyond, as he carried the wisdom and love of the garden with him, sharing its beauty and serenity with all who crossed his path.

And so, as the sun set each evening, casting its warm, golden light over the thriving landscape of the garden, Edward would pause and take a moment to offer his thanks—for the simple joy of tending to the earth, for the profound beauty of nature's delicate balance, and for the sanctuary of peace and solace that he had found within the gentle embrace of his beloved garden.

The Weaver's Melody

Amelia stood before her loom, her hands poised above the wooden frame as she prepared to begin her day's work. The room was filled with the soft, diffused light of morning, casting a warm glow on the vibrant threads that lay waiting to be woven into a tapestry of intricate patterns and designs. It was in these quiet moments, as she surrendered herself to the gentle rhythm of the loom, that Amelia found solace and comfort in the familiar dance of warp and weft.

With a deep breath, Amelia began to weave, her skilled hands moving with grace and precision as she guided the shuttle through the threads, creating a mesmerizing pattern that seemed to unfold like a living, breathing work of art. The loom itself seemed to sing as she worked, its wooden frame humming a soothing melody that resonated through the room, enveloping Amelia in a cocoon of sound and motion.

As the hours passed and the tapestry took shape, Amelia found her thoughts wandering through the landscape of her life, her memories unspooling like the threads that she so skillfully wove together. Each strand seemed to hold its own unique story, a vibrant thread in the tapestry of her experiences that spanned the years of her life.

She recalled the first time she had sat before a loom, her small, trembling hands guided by the gentle touch of her grandmother, a skilled weaver in her own right. It was from her that Amelia had learned the secrets of the craft, the ancient techniques and patterns passed down through generations of women who had found solace and purpose in the rhythmic dance of the loom.

As Amelia's thoughts drifted, she found herself reliving the many joys and sorrows that had marked her journey, each one adding depth and color to the tapestry of her life. She remembered the laughter and tears, the triumphs and heartaches, and the countless moments of quiet reflection that had shaped her into the woman she had become.

Through it all, the loom had been her constant companion, a source of solace and comfort in times of turmoil and a wellspring of inspiration and creativity in moments of joy. The rhythm of the loom seemed to echo the beat of her heart, a steady, comforting presence that anchored her to the world and provided a sense of purpose and connection.

As the day wore on and the tapestry grew, Amelia became more and more absorbed in the delicate interplay of threads and colors, each one a testament to the beauty of life's ever-changing tapestry. She marveled at the intricate patterns that seemed to emerge, as if by magic, from the simple act of weaving, and she found herself lost in the silent poetry of the loom's melody.

In these moments of quiet contemplation, Amelia discovered a profound sense of peace, a connection to something greater than herself that transcended the boundaries of her small, sunlit room. She understood that in the gentle, rhythmic dance of the loom, she was not only creating a work of art but also weaving a new strand in the tapestry of her own life, adding depth and beauty to the rich, vibrant fabric of her existence.

As the sun began to set, casting its golden light on the finished tapestry that now adorned the loom, Amelia stepped back to admire her work. The intricate patterns and vibrant colors seemed to dance before her eyes, a visual symphony that spoke of the love and care she had poured into every stitch.

With a sense of quiet satisfaction, Amelia carefully removed the tapestry from the loom, her fingers tracing the delicate patterns and textures that told the story of her day's labor. She knew that in the gentle, rhythmic melody of the loom, she had found not only solace and comfort but also a powerful connection to the timeless beauty of life's ever-changing tapestry.

As Amelia folded the tapestry and placed it in a wooden chest filled with her other creations, she felt a deep sense of gratitude for the simple joy of weaving and for the many lessons and memories that her beloved loom had brought her. She understood that each thread, each intricate pattern, held a piece of her own story and a testament to the enduring power of love, creativity, and self-expression.

As the last rays of sunlight faded from the room, Amelia took a moment to offer her thanks—for the gift of her grandmother's wisdom and guidance, for the solace and inspiration she found in the gentle dance of the loom, and for the beautiful tapestry of life that continued to unfold around her.

With a peaceful heart, Amelia tidied her workspace and closed the door behind her, the melody of the loom still echoing in her ears, a soothing lullaby that carried her through the evening and into the welcoming embrace of the night. In the quiet moments before sleep claimed her, Amelia knew that she had found something truly special in the simple act of weaving, a sanctuary of peace and serenity that she would carry with her, always, as she continued her journey through life's ever-changing landscape.

The Lighthouse Keeper's Solitude

James stepped out onto the balcony of the lighthouse, a gentle breeze ruffling his hair as he gazed out at the vast expanse of the ocean before him. From his isolated post at the edge of the world, he watched as the water stretched out to meet the horizon, an ever-changing canvas of blues and grays that seemed to mirror the moods of the sky above.

As the lighthouse keeper, James had grown accustomed to the solitude and quiet of his life on the rocky shore, a world far removed from the hustle and bustle of the city he had left behind. In the rhythmic ebb and flow of the tides, he found a sense of peace and comfort that had eluded him for so long, a balm for the weary soul that had led him to this remote outpost at the edge of the sea.

In the mornings, James would often take long walks along the shoreline, breathing in the salty air and listening to the calls of the seabirds as they swooped and soared above the waves. The steady rhythm of the surf and the cries of the gulls seemed to be the only constants in this ever-shifting landscape, a reassuring reminder of the world's enduring beauty and the timeless ebb and flow of life.

As he explored the craggy cliffs and hidden coves that surrounded the lighthouse, James discovered a wealth of natural wonders that he had never known existed. He marveled at the delicate beauty of the tide pools, teeming with life and color, and found solace in the quiet majesty of the towering sea cliffs that guarded the coast.

With each passing day, James felt more and more at home in this wild and untamed landscape, his spirit renewed by the raw power and beauty of the ocean and the solitude that his life as a lighthouse keeper provided.

As the sun began its slow descent towards the horizon, casting its golden light on the water's surface, James felt a familiar sense of anticipation begin to build. It was in these twilight hours that the lighthouse truly came alive, its powerful beacon of light cutting through the darkness to guide sailors safely home.

With practiced ease, James began the process of lighting the lighthouse's lamp, carefully tending to the delicate mechanisms that powered the great beacon. As the first flicker of light began to dance on the water's surface, he felt a surge of pride and satisfaction, knowing that his work was not only a testament to his own dedication but also a lifeline for those who traveled the treacherous seas.

As the night wore on and the lighthouse cast its steady, reassuring light across the waves, James found himself lost in the mesmerizing dance of illumination on the water. The shifting patterns of light and shadow seemed to take on a life of their own, a visual symphony that played out on the vast, dark stage of the ocean.

In these quiet moments of solitude, James found a sense of connection to the natural world that he had never known before. He marveled at the raw, untamed beauty of the sea, its moods as varied and complex as his own, and the delicate balance of life that thrived within its depths.

He watched as the moon rose, casting its silvery glow on the water and illuminating the way for the countless creatures that called the ocean their home. In the gentle lapping of the waves against the shore, he heard the whispered secrets of the sea, stories of adventure and love, of tragedy and triumph, carried on the currents that crisscrossed the globe.

As he stood watch over the coastline, James found solace in the knowledge that he was part of a long and storied tradition, a lineage of lighthouse keepers who had braved the isolation and the elements to ensure the safety of those who ventured out into the unforgiving seas. He felt a deep sense of responsibility and purpose, knowing that his work was not only important but also a vital lifeline for countless lives.

During the day, James would often spend his time tending to the lighthouse and its grounds, performing routine maintenance tasks and ensuring that everything was in working order. The rhythmic, methodical nature of his work brought him a sense of calm and satisfaction, a welcome respite from the chaos and uncertainty of the world beyond.

As the seasons changed and the weather turned, James found himself adapting to the rhythms of his new life, learning to appreciate the beauty and mystery of the world around him. He watched in awe as storms raged across the ocean, the waves crashing against the cliffs with a primal force that was both terrifying and awe-inspiring.

In the quiet aftermath of the storm, he would venture out to survey the damage and marvel at the resilience of the natural world, the way it seemed to bounce back from even the most violent of upheavals. And as the sun emerged from behind the clouds and the world began to heal, he felt a deep sense of gratitude for the solace and sanctuary that his life as a lighthouse keeper had provided.

As the years passed and the world continued to change around him, James found that his connection to the ocean and the solitude of his life at the lighthouse only deepened, a source of comfort and strength that he carried with him always.

In the quiet moments between his work and his solitary contemplation, he found that he had become a part of the landscape itself, his spirit woven into the fabric of the cliffs and the sea, his presence a constant and reassuring presence on the edge of the vast, untamed ocean.

With the first rays of the sun breaking over the horizon, James extinguished the lighthouse lamp and prepared to begin another day, his heart filled with the knowledge that he was not only the guardian of the lighthouse but also a witness to the enduring beauty and mystery of the ocean's ever-changing tapestry.

As he stood on the balcony, watching as the world awoke around him, he knew that he had found something truly special in his life as a lighthouse keeper. In the solitude and serenity of his isolated post, he had discovered a world of wonder and beauty that he would carry with him always, a source of comfort and inspiration that would see him through the darkest nights and guide him safely home.

And as the sun climbed higher in the sky and the world continued its endless dance of light and shadow, James felt a deep sense of peace and contentment, knowing that he had found his place in the world, a refuge from the storm and a sanctuary where he could finally be at one with the ever-changing beauty of the sea.

Sunset Stroll

As the warm glow of the setting sun began to paint the sky with brilliant hues of orange and red, I laced up my comfortable walking shoes and stepped out of my front door, eager to embark on my evening stroll. With each step, I felt the day's worries and stresses begin to melt away, replaced by a sense of peace and tranquility that only the gentle embrace of nature could provide.

The familiar path wound its way through a quiet park, the soft rustling of leaves and the gentle cooing of birds providing a soothing soundtrack for my journey. With each step, I felt more connected to the world around me, more in tune with the subtle beauty of the natural world.

As I walked, I took the time to appreciate the myriad of sensory experiences that enveloped me. The earthy scent of damp soil rose from the ground, mingling with the sweet fragrance of blossoming flowers. The gentle breeze whispered through the trees, carrying with it the faint laughter of children playing in the distance.

I paused for a moment to run my fingers through the velvety petals of a nearby flower, marveling at the delicate beauty and intricate structure of the bloom. The vibrant colors seemed to come alive beneath my touch, a living testament to the power and wonder of nature's creations.

My eyes were drawn to the vibrant colors of the setting sun, the sky a canvas of fiery reds and golds that seemed to set the world alight with their brilliance. As I continued along the path, the colors shifted and deepened, evolving into a rich tapestry of purples and blues as the day began its slow surrender to the encroaching night.

As the sun dipped lower in the sky, casting long, dappled shadows across the path, I marveled at the delicate interplay of light and shadow, the way the world seemed to transform before my eyes as the day drew to a close. The air grew cooler, a refreshing contrast to the warmth of the sun on my skin, and I felt a sense of peace and contentment wash over me, a quiet appreciation for the simple beauty of the world around me.

I wandered off the path for a moment, drawn to a small grove of trees that seemed to beckon with their outstretched branches. The leaves rustled softly overhead as I walked beneath the canopy, the sunlight filtering through the foliage and casting a verdant, dappled light on the forest floor. I closed my eyes for a moment, allowing the sounds of the rustling leaves and the distant call of birds to envelop me, a soothing lullaby that seemed to echo the slow, rhythmic beating of my heart.

As I continued my walk, I noticed the changing texture of the ground beneath my feet, the soft, yielding earth giving way to the crunch of gravel and the cool, smooth surface of a paved pathway. With each step, I felt more grounded, more connected to the world around me, as though the very earth itself was reaching out to embrace me and welcome me home.

As twilight approached and the first stars began to appear in the deepening sky, I found my footsteps growing slower, more deliberate, as I allowed myself to become fully immersed in the sensory experience of the world around me. The soft, muted colors of dusk enveloped the landscape, casting everything in a gentle, ethereal glow that seemed to exist somewhere between reality and the realm of dreams.

I paused for a moment on a small wooden bridge, leaning against the railing and allowing my gaze to be drawn to the rippling surface of the water below. The fading light danced on the water, the liquid surface reflecting the colors of the sky and creating a mesmerizing, ever-changing pattern that seemed to echo the ebb and flow of my own thoughts and emotions. I closed my eyes and listened to the gentle lapping of the water against the bridge's supports, the soothing sound washing over me like a balm for my weary soul.

As the sky grew darker and the world around me became cloaked in the velvety embrace of night, I noticed the subtle changes in the sounds and scents that filled the air. The sweet, floral perfume of the blossoming flowers gave way to the earthy aroma of dew-kissed grass, while the chirping of birds was replaced by the soft, rhythmic chorus of crickets and the distant hoot of an owl.

I continued my stroll, drawn by the allure of the path as it meandered through the park, past small ponds and clusters of trees that seemed to whisper their ancient secrets in the stillness of the night. I allowed my hands to brush gently against the cool, rough bark of the trees as I passed, feeling a sense of connection to the timeless wisdom and serenity that seemed to emanate from their very core.

As the moon began to rise, casting a silvery glow over the landscape, I found myself standing at the edge of a wide, open field, the tall grass swaying gently in the evening breeze. The world around me seemed to shimmer and dance in the moonlight, the delicate interplay of shadow and light casting a spell of enchantment over the scene.

I took a deep breath, filling my lungs with the crisp, cool air, and felt a sense of awe and wonder at the beauty of the world around me. I felt as though I was standing on the threshold of a dream, the boundary between the waking world and the realm of sleep, and I knew that the memory of this peaceful, sensory-rich stroll would stay with me long after I returned to the comfort of my home.

As I made my way back along the path, the night sky above me filled with a multitude of twinkling stars, I was filled with a deep sense of gratitude and appreciation for the simple, profound beauty of the natural world. I knew that I would carry the memory of this sunset stroll with me always, a reminder of the solace and serenity that could be found in the quiet, unassuming moments of life, and the power of nature to heal and restore the weary soul.

The Timekeeper's Clock

In the quiet solitude of his small, cluttered workshop, the clockmaker carefully examined the antique timepiece that lay before him on the workbench. Its intricate inner workings were a testament to the skill and artistry of a long-forgotten craftsman, and he felt a deep sense of reverence and responsibility as he set about the delicate task of restoring the clock to its former glory.

The soft, muted light of the workshop cast a warm glow over the myriad of tools and components that surrounded him, each piece a part of the complex puzzle that was the inner workings of the timepiece. With a steady hand and a keen eye, he carefully disassembled the clock, laying out each individual part with precision and care.

As he worked, he found solace in the rhythmic ticking of the other clocks that filled the room, their steady, hypnotic cadence a comforting reminder of the passage of time and the fleeting nature of each moment. He felt a sense of kinship with the timepieces, each one a living, breathing testament to the power of time and the beauty of the moments that make up our lives.

With each gear, spring, and pinion that he cleaned and polished, he felt the weight of the world slipping away, replaced by a sense of calm focus and quiet determination. The simple, repetitive tasks of restoration provided a welcome respite from the chaos and uncertainty of the world outside, and he found himself immersed in a state of tranquil mindfulness as he worked.

As the hours passed, the timekeeper's hands moved deftly over the intricate components, the steady rhythm of his work mirroring the measured ticking of the clocks that surrounded him. Each small, precise movement brought the antique timepiece one step closer to its former glory, the delicate interplay of gears and springs slowly coming back to life beneath his skilled touch.

In the silence of the workshop, he allowed his mind to wander, reflecting on the passage of time and the countless moments that had slipped through his fingers like grains of sand. He thought of the hands that had crafted the timepiece, the lives that it had touched, and the moments it had marked with its quiet, unassuming presence.

As the restoration neared completion, he marveled at the beauty and intricacy of the clock's inner workings, the delicate dance of gears and springs that marked the passage of each moment. He thought of the countless hours that had been poured into the creation of the timepiece, the skill and dedication of the craftsman who had brought it to life, and the legacy of time and love that it represented.

Finally, with a gentle, reverent touch, he placed the last piece of the puzzle, the delicate hands of the clock, back into position. As he wound the key and set the time, he felt a sense of pride and satisfaction wash over him, a quiet appreciation for the simple, profound beauty of the work he had just completed.

With the restored timepiece now ticking steadily beside him, he allowed himself a moment of quiet contemplation, his thoughts turning to the fleeting nature of time and the importance of cherishing each and every moment. The gentle, rhythmic ticking of the clock seemed to echo the beating of his own heart, a constant, comforting reminder of the passage of time and the beauty of the moments that make up our lives.

As the day drew to a close, and the soft light of the setting sun filtered through the workshop's windows, casting a warm, golden glow over the room, he stood back and admired the beauty of the antique timepiece, its delicate hands tracing an eternal dance across the face of the clock. He knew that the restoration of this beautiful, intricate work of art was more than just a testament to his own skill and dedication; it was a tribute to the timeless art of clockmaking and a celebration of the countless moments that made up the rich tapestry of life.

As he listened to the rhythmic ticking of the restored clock, he felt a deep sense of connection to the past, present, and future, the unbroken chain of moments that bound together the lives of all who had been touched by the timepiece's quiet, unassuming presence. He thought of the countless others who had stood before the clock, their lives marked by the steady, unyielding passage of time, and he felt a profound sense of gratitude for the opportunity to play a small part in the ongoing story of this beautiful, timeless creation.

In the quiet solitude of his workshop, surrounded by the soft, hypnotic ticking of the clocks, he found a sense of peace and contentment that seemed to transcend the boundaries of time and space. Each beat of the clock's heart seemed to whisper a message of hope and renewal, a reminder that even as time slipped away, there was beauty and meaning to be found in the simple, unassuming moments of life.

As the shadows grew longer and the day began to surrender to the encroaching darkness of night, the clockmaker allowed himself a final moment of quiet reflection, the restored timepiece standing proudly beside him as a testament to the power of dedication, craftsmanship, and the enduring beauty of time itself. With a gentle smile, he reached out and touched the clock's smooth, polished surface, feeling the steady pulse of its rhythmic ticking beneath his fingertips, and knew that he had succeeded in creating something truly extraordinary.

With a sense of quiet satisfaction, he turned off the workshop lights, leaving the restored timepiece to continue its eternal dance in the soft, comforting darkness. As he made his way to the door, the gentle, rhythmic ticking of the clocks seemed to follow him, a quiet, comforting reminder of the beauty and wonder to be found in the simple, unassuming moments of life, and the power of time to heal, restore, and reveal the extraordinary in the ordinary.

A Cup of Serenity

As twilight descended, casting a gentle veil of darkness over the world outside, I found myself standing in the cozy warmth of my kitchen, the soft glow of the overhead light casting a welcoming aura over the room. The day had been long and filled with the usual hustle and bustle, but now, in the quiet stillness of the evening, I had the chance to unwind and savor the simple pleasure of a warm cup of tea.

With practiced ease, I filled the kettle with water and set it on the stove, the comforting sound of the flame igniting beneath it bringing an instant sense of calm. As I waited for the water to heat, I gazed out the window, watching as the first few drops of rain began to fall, leaving delicate trails on the glass that shimmered in the fading light.

I selected my favorite tea blend from the cupboard, a soothing mix of chamomile, lavender, and lemon balm that never failed to bring a sense of peace and tranquility to my weary soul. As the kettle began to whistle, I carefully poured the steaming water over the tea leaves, watching as the rich, golden liquid began to fill my favorite mug. I marveled at the subtle shift in color, as the water transformed into a calming elixir, the scent of the blend already beginning to fill the air with its soothing aroma.

With my warm cup of serenity in hand, I made my way to the living room, settling into the plush embrace of my favorite armchair. The soft patter of rain against the windowpane seemed to blend seamlessly with the quiet hiss of the steam rising from my tea, creating a symphony of soothing sounds that filled the room.

The gentle flickering of candlelight cast a warm, comforting glow over the room, creating a sanctuary from the world outside. The flickering flames cast shadows that seemed to dance gracefully across the walls, adding to the sense of tranquility and peace that enveloped me. The soft, plush cushions of my armchair cradled my body, allowing me to sink into a state of complete relaxation, free from the worries and stresses that had accumulated throughout the day.

As I took my first sip, I closed my eyes and allowed the warmth of the tea to spread through my body, the fragrant blend of herbs and flowers working its magic on my senses. The delicate, calming flavors seemed to carry me away, transporting me to a place of quiet repose, a world where the chaos of everyday life was replaced by the simple, profound beauty of nature.

With each sip, I felt my connection to the world outside grow stronger, the gentle rhythm of the raindrops on the windowpane reminding me of the power of nature to heal and restore. I allowed my thoughts to drift like the raindrops, following their meandering path as they traced intricate patterns on the glass.

The sound of the rain seemed to envelop the room, creating a soothing white noise that drowned out the distant hum of the world outside. I let my mind wander through the memories of past rainy days, the feeling of safety and warmth as I watched the world outside from the comfort of my home. Each memory brought with it a sense of peace, a reminder of the simple, unassuming beauty that could be found in even the most ordinary moments.

As the rain continued to fall, I found myself lost in the beauty of the moment, the soothing warmth of the tea in my hands and the hypnotic sound of the raindrops against the windowpane creating a sense of perfect harmony. The world outside seemed to recede into the background, replaced by the quiet, unassuming presence of the rain and the comforting embrace of my steaming cup of tea.

As I took the last sip from my mug, I felt a deep sense of gratitude and contentment wash over me, a quiet appreciation for the simple pleasure of a warm cup of tea and the calming effect of nature. I knew that this moment, this quiet evening spent in the company of the rain and the warmth of my favorite tea, would stay with me long after the rain had stopped and the day had given way to the promise of a new dawn.

With a gentle sigh, I rose from my armchair and carried my empty mug back to the kitchen, pausing to gaze out the window once more. The rain was falling more heavily now, the droplets creating ripples in the puddles that had formed on the ground outside. The sight of the rain-soaked world beyond the glass seemed to amplify the warmth and comfort of my home, a reminder of the sanctuary I had created for myself within the walls of my house.

I placed the empty mug in the sink, watching as the last few raindrops fell from the sky and disappeared into the night. I took a moment to breathe in the lingering scent of the tea, the soothing aroma a reminder of the peace and serenity I had found within the walls of my home, away from the chaos and noise of the world outside.

As I turned off the light and made my way to bed, I carried with me the memory of this quiet evening, a gentle reminder of the solace and serenity to be found in the simple, unassuming moments of life. The soft patter of rain continued to echo through the house as I drifted off to sleep, a lullaby that seemed to sing of the beauty and wonder of the world, of the magic that could be found in the quiet spaces between the raindrops and the comforting warmth of a steaming cup of tea.

The night passed peacefully, the rain acting as a soothing balm to the weary soul, and when morning came, the world outside seemed renewed, washed clean by the gentle embrace of the rain. As I awoke and made my way back to the kitchen, the memory of the quiet evening spent with my cup of serenity remained, a gentle reminder of the beauty and peace that could be found in tiny moments, and the power of nature to heal, restore, and bring solace to even the most weary of souls.

Watercolor Dreams

I stood in my small, sunlit studio, my brush poised delicately above the palette, the bristles dripping with a mixture of azure and cerulean hues. The soft afternoon light filtered through the gauzy curtains, casting a warm glow over the room and illuminating the blank canvas before me. With each breath, I inhaled the faint scent of dampened paper and watercolors, a subtle reminder of the creative journey I was about to embark upon.

Gently, I touched the brush to the canvas, watching as the pigments bled and merged, creating a sky of infinite shades and depth. I reveled in the process, my attention focused on each individual color as it swirled and combined with the others. The sensation of the brush on the paper was soothing, each stroke a delicate dance that left a trail of subtle hues in its wake.

As the sky began to take shape, I moved on to the landscape below. I mixed a deep, rich green, experimenting with the balance of water and pigment to achieve the perfect consistency. I carefully applied it to the canvas, creating lush hills and valleys that seemed to roll and undulate beneath the vibrant sky. The colors continued to blend and transform as they dried, a living testament to the dynamic nature of watercolors.

I began to layer in more colors, adding depth and complexity to the scene before me. I experimented with varying shades of green, capturing the play of light and shadow across the landscape as the sun dipped lower in the sky. I allowed the colors to mingle and mix on the canvas, watching in fascination as they transformed into new, unexpected hues.

My attention then turned to the trees that dotted the landscape. I carefully mixed a series of earthy browns and greens, adjusting the ratios until I was satisfied with the results. I painted in the trunks and branches, then used a wet-on-wet technique to create the soft, ethereal foliage. The result was a dreamy, impressionistic forest that seemed to whisper of hidden secrets and quiet, serene moments.

With the landscape complete, I turned my focus to the foreground, where I envisioned a quiet stream meandering through the scene. I mixed a series of blues and greens, striving to create the perfect shade to convey the sense of cool, clear water. I carefully painted in the stream, allowing the colors to blend and flow like the water it represented.

As I worked, I continued to experiment with different techniques and color combinations, embracing the unpredictable nature of watercolors. I discovered the beauty in allowing the colors to flow and blend freely, giving up a measure of control in order to achieve a more organic, natural result. The process was both calming and invigorating, each new discovery fueling my passion for the medium.

I paused to step back and assess my work, taking note of any areas that required further attention or adjustment. I carefully added in small details, such as the delicate blades of grass that lined the stream or the subtle play of light on the leaves of the trees. With each additional layer and detail, the painting became more vivid and lifelike, an intricate tapestry of colors and textures that drew the eye and captured the imagination.

As I continued to work, the afternoon wore on, the golden light of the sun gradually giving way to the soft, muted hues of twilight. The changing light brought new depth and dimension to the colors on the canvas, the shifting shadows and highlights adding a sense of movement and life to the scene.

Eventually, the sun dipped below the horizon, and the room was bathed in the gentle glow of twilight. I set my brush down, taking a moment to appreciate the beauty of the finished painting. The colors seemed to shimmer and dance, the delicate watercolor landscape a testament to the power of art and the process of creation. The canvas was a world unto itself, a tranquil haven that invited the viewer to escape the chaos of everyday life and find solace in the soothing embrace of nature.

As I cleaned my brushes and packed away my supplies, my thoughts lingered on the hours spent immersed in the world of watercolors. The experience had been a meditative one, my focus on the colors and the act of painting serving as a balm for my restless mind. In the quiet solitude of my studio, I had found a sense of inner peace and contentment that only the act of creation could provide.

With a deep sense of satisfaction, I turned off the lights and left my studio, the soft glow of the moonlight casting a final, ethereal light on my completed painting. I carried with me the memories of the afternoon spent exploring the delicate world of watercolors, a reminder of the serenity and calm that could be found in the simple act of bringing a vision to life on canvas.

As I lay in bed that night, the images and colors from the painting danced through my mind, lulling me into a state of peaceful relaxation. I drifted off to sleep with thoughts of azure skies, verdant hills, and the gentle lullaby of the stream, the watercolor dreams a soothing balm for my weary soul. I knew that the memories of that afternoon would stay with me, a reminder of the healing power of art and the beauty that lay in the quiet moments of life, waiting to be discovered and cherished.

Stargazer's Solace

Alex stepped out onto the dew-kissed grass of the backyard, the cool night air wrapping around him like a comforting embrace. Above him, the night sky stretched out in all its splendor, a vast canvas painted with the glimmering light of distant stars. The quiet hush of the evening enveloped him, and he felt the tension in his body begin to dissipate as he gazed upward in awe.

The soft glow of the moon bathed the landscape in silver light, casting long, ethereal shadows that danced and swayed with the gentle rustling of leaves in the breeze. In the distance, the rhythmic chorus of crickets and the gentle hoots of a pair of owls provided a soothing soundtrack to the night's celestial display.

With his trusty telescope by his side, Alex slowly scanned the heavens, his eyes seeking out familiar constellations and celestial landmarks. The sight of the Big Dipper, its stars shining like beacons in the darkness, brought a smile to his face, as it always did. He marveled at the thought that the patterns he saw in the sky had been recognized and revered by countless generations before him, a testament to the enduring allure of the cosmos.

As Alex continued to explore the night sky, he stumbled upon the radiant glow of Jupiter, its presence a reminder of the vastness of the universe and the seemingly infinite number of worlds that lay hidden within it. He marveled at the thought of the swirling storms and tumultuous winds that raged across the surface of the gas giant, a stark contrast to the serene beauty it projected from afar.

Alex trained his telescope on the distant speck of light, his heart pounding with anticipation as the image came into focus. There, suspended in the inky blackness of space, was the unmistakable sight of Jupiter's cloud bands and its four largest moons, strung out like celestial pearls against the velvety backdrop. He felt a shiver of excitement course through him as he considered the enormity of the sight before him, the knowledge that he was gazing upon another world, millions of miles away from his own.

With each celestial body Alex observed, he felt his connection to the cosmos deepen, the vast expanse of the universe both humbling and awe-inspiring. The sight of the glittering stars and distant planets seemed to put the worries and stresses of daily life into perspective, a gentle reminder of the small and fleeting nature of our existence in the grand scheme of things.

Alex turned his telescope towards the distant spiral arms of the Milky Way, the shimmering band of stars a testament to the vastness and complexity of our galaxy. The delicate dance of stars across the sky served as a reminder that, despite the immensity of the universe, there was a sense of order and harmony that pervaded its expanse.

As the hours passed, Alex became further entranced by the celestial wonders that filled his view. He shifted his gaze to the Andromeda galaxy, a hazy smudge of light that was, in reality, a swirling mass of billions of stars, gas, and dust. The thought that he was witnessing the light from a galaxy over two million light-years away left him in awe, marveling at the incredible distances that separated the stars and the immense scale of the universe itself.

The constellations seemed to dance around him, their patterns telling ancient stories of heroes, gods, and mythical creatures. Alex felt a connection to the generations of stargazers who had come before him, their eyes lifted towards the same sky, seeking solace and inspiration in the mysteries of the cosmos.

As the night progressed, the stars seemed to grow brighter, the darkness of the sky deepening to a rich, velvety black. The air had become crisp, and Alex wrapped himself in a warm blanket, his breath visible in the cool night air. The quiet stillness of the night enveloped him, a sense of peace and tranquility settling over him as he continued his celestial journey.

Eventually, the first hints of dawn began to creep over the horizon, casting a soft, golden light on the landscape. The stars began to fade as the sun made its slow ascent, signaling the end of another night spent beneath the vast canopy of the cosmos.

Alex reluctantly packed away his telescope, his eyes lingering on the sky as the last stars winked out of sight. As he made his way back inside, he carried with him the sense of wonder and serenity that the night sky had bestowed upon him, a reminder of the beauty and majesty of the universe that lay just beyond his doorstep.

The night's stargazing had been a balm to his soul, a moment of quiet introspection in the midst of a chaotic world. As he settled into bed, Alex closed his eyes, the memories of the celestial wonders he had witnessed lulling him into a peaceful, restful sleep.

Nature's Symphony

As the morning sun crept over the horizon, casting its warm, golden light through the trees, James eagerly laced up his hiking boots, preparing for his favorite weekend ritual – a leisurely walk through the nearby forest. He cherished these moments of solitude, an opportunity to escape the hustle and bustle of city life and immerse himself in the soothing embrace of nature.

James set out, the damp, earthy scent of the forest floor filling his nostrils as he took his first steps on the winding path that led him deeper into the woods. The air was cool and fresh, still carrying the lingering traces of the previous night's rain. As he walked, he could feel the dampness beneath his feet, the soil springing back with each step, creating a satisfying cushioning sensation.

As he ventured further into the forest, James became keenly aware of the multitude of sounds that filled the air around him. The leaves rustled gently above his head, their whispered conversations carried on the soft, playful breeze. The swaying branches of the trees created a delicate symphony of creaks and groans, a testament to their resilience and strength.

Birdsong filled the air, a cacophony of melodies that seemed to celebrate the beauty and majesty of the forest. The fluting call of a thrush echoed through the canopy, its sweet, lilting notes a welcome companion on James's journey. High above, the excited chatter of squirrels could be heard as they leaped from branch to branch, their energetic acrobatics a source of endless fascination.

As James continued along the path, the sound of a babbling brook reached his ears, a gentle, rhythmic accompaniment to the forest's chorus. The soothing sound of the water drew him closer, and he soon found himself standing on the bank of a crystal-clear stream. The water tumbled gracefully over smooth, rounded stones, its melodious flow a balm to his weary soul.

He took a moment to pause and listen, the music of the stream intermingling with the chorus of birds and the rustling leaves to create a symphony that seemed to speak directly to his heart. The quiet gurgling of the water, the gentle splashes as it flowed over rocks and fallen branches, lulled him into a state of deep relaxation, his mind unburdened by the concerns and stresses of everyday life.

James closed his eyes and allowed the sounds of the forest to envelop him, the rich tapestry of auditory sensations weaving a cocoon of tranquility around him. The distant drumming of a woodpecker at work resonated through the air, its rhythmic tapping a reminder of the intricate web of life that thrived within the forest.

As he continued on his walk, James found himself drawn to the rustle of leaves underfoot, the satisfying crunch as he stepped on fallen twigs and crisp foliage. The sounds of the forest seemed to grow more complex and layered with each step he took, as if nature was revealing its secrets to him, one note at a time.

The forest floor was a symphony of its own, the soft rustling of unseen creatures and the gentle patter of raindrops falling from the leaves above adding to the rich auditory landscape. Each sound seemed to have its place, each note a vital component of the forest's song.

As James ventured further, the wind picked up, adding its own voice to the chorus. The trees swayed and danced, their branches rubbing against one another, creating an ever-changing melody that seemed to echo the ebb and flow of the world beyond the forest's edge.

He felt a profound sense of connection to the world around him, the sounds of the forest serving as a reminder of the intricate balance of life and the interconnectedness of all living things. The forest's symphony was a testament to the beauty of the natural world, a celebration of the delicate harmony that existed within its boundaries.

As the sun began its slow descent towards the horizon, the sounds of the forest began to shift, giving way to a new chorus of nocturnal voices. The call of an owl pierced the twilight, its haunting melody a reminder of the mysteries that lay hidden in the shadows. The soft, ghostly rustle of bats taking flight filled the air, their silent, graceful movements a captivating sight against the darkening sky.

James reluctantly turned back, retracing his steps along the path as the final rays of sunlight filtered through the trees, casting long, dappled shadows on the forest floor. The sounds of the forest seemed to take on a more subdued, introspective quality as the day drew to a close, a gentle lullaby that seemed to soothe the soul.

As he made his way home, James felt a deep sense of gratitude for the time he had spent within the forest's embrace, the symphony of sounds that had accompanied him on his journey a balm to his weary spirit. The forest had once again provided him with a sanctuary, a place to escape the pressures of the outside world and find solace in the beauty and wonder of nature.

As he closed the door behind him, the sounds of the forest still echoing in his ears, James knew that he would carry the memories of his walk with him, the gentle symphony of the woods a reminder of the peace and tranquility that could be found in the simplest of pleasures. And as he drifted off to sleep that night, the soothing lullaby of the forest played softly in his mind, a testament to the enduring power of nature's symphony.

The Book Nook

It was a cool, gray afternoon, the kind that seemed to call for a warm blanket and a good book. Liam had been looking forward to this all week – a quiet moment to escape the demands of his hectic life and indulge in his favorite pastime. As he crossed the threshold of his favorite room in the house, his eyes lit up with anticipation. This was his sanctuary, his personal book nook, filled with shelves of well-loved novels and an inviting reading chair nestled by the window.

The walls of the room were lined with bookshelves, each one teeming with stories waiting to be discovered. The wooden floor was adorned with a plush, patterned rug that added a touch of warmth and color to the cozy space. A small side table stood beside the reading chair, a place for a steaming cup of tea or a flickering candle to further enhance the soothing atmosphere.

Liam took a deep breath, the familiar scent of paper and ink filling his nostrils, bringing with it a profound sense of comfort and nostalgia. He perused the shelves, his fingers lightly brushing the spines of the books as he searched for the perfect companion for the afternoon. It was an old favorite that caught his eye, a worn copy of a cherished novel that had seen him through many a rainy day.

With a contented sigh, Liam settled into the plush reading chair, a warm, cozy blanket draped across his lap. The cushion seemed to envelop him, offering a gentle embrace as he opened the book to the first page. The familiar words greeted him like old friends, the opening lines as comforting as a well-worn quilt.

As Liam began to read, he felt the stresses and worries of the day slowly slipping away, replaced by the gentle magic of the written word. The prose flowed like a soothing melody, each sentence a gentle caress that seemed to lull him into a state of deep relaxation. The world outside faded into the background, the dull murmur of the rain against the windowpane a distant whisper compared to the vibrant, captivating world within the pages of the book.

The characters came to life before his eyes, their hopes and dreams, triumphs and sorrows unfolding with each turn of the page. Liam felt a kinship with these fictional beings, their stories resonating with his own experiences, providing a sense of connection and understanding that transcended the boundaries of ink and paper.

He became immersed in the landscape of the story, the author's descriptive language painting vivid scenes in his mind. The rustling of leaves in a dense forest, the gentle lapping of waves on a moonlit beach – each setting was rendered with such detail and care that Liam felt as though he was truly there, experiencing these places alongside the characters.

As the hours passed, the soft glow of the reading lamp cast a warm, golden light on the pages, the dancing shadows on the walls creating an atmosphere of peace and tranquility. The gentle sound of the rain outside seemed to provide the perfect accompaniment to the story, its rhythmic patter serving as a reminder of the soothing power of nature.

The plot unfolded at a leisurely pace, allowing Liam to savor each moment, each nuance of the narrative. He delighted in the author's turns of phrase, the way they could capture the essence of an emotion or a memory with just a few carefully chosen words. The dialogue between the characters felt natural and engaging, each exchange revealing new layers of depth and complexity.

As the afternoon gave way to evening, and the last page was turned, Liam felt a sense of contentment and fulfillment that only a truly great book could provide. He closed the cover gently, a smile tugging at the corners of his lips as he took a moment to savor the experience he had just shared with the characters and the world within the pages. The rain had tapered off, leaving a hushed silence in its wake, as if the world outside was holding its breath, allowing him to fully absorb the story's lingering echoes.

Liam glanced around his book nook, his eyes taking in the familiar surroundings with a renewed sense of appreciation. The soft, warm glow of the reading lamp, the comforting embrace of the plush chair, and the shelves lined with countless other literary adventures – each element contributed to the creation of this haven of serenity and introspection.

He felt grateful for the opportunity to escape, even if just for a few hours, into the enchanting world of literature. It was a rare gift to be able to lose oneself so completely in a story, to become so thoroughly immersed in the lives of the characters and the vivid landscapes they inhabited. These moments of quiet reflection and connection with the written word were a balm to his soul, providing a respite from the relentless pace of daily life.

With a contented sigh, Liam carefully returned the book to its place on the shelf, giving the spine an affectionate pat as if to thank it for the journey they had shared. As he stepped away from the bookcase, he felt a renewed sense of calm and tranquility, the lingering magic of the story continuing to resonate within him.

As he left the sanctuary of his book nook, Liam carried with him the echoes of the world he had just explored, the characters and their experiences etched into his memory. He knew that the next time the world seemed too much to bear, he could return to this cozy refuge, pick up another book, and once again lose himself in the gentle, soothing embrace of the written word.

Whispers of Winter

Sophia stood at the edge of the snow-covered forest, the morning light casting a soft, ethereal glow on the pristine landscape. The world seemed to be holding its breath, the hushed silence of the snow-draped trees and the frozen ground beneath her feet creating an atmosphere of stillness and tranquility. She wrapped her scarf a little tighter around her neck and took a deep breath, the crisp, cold air filling her lungs as she stepped onto the path that led into the heart of the woods.

The snow crunched softly beneath her boots, each step leaving a fresh set of prints on the untouched white blanket that lay before her. The branches of the trees overhead were laden with snow, their delicate, lacy patterns weaving an intricate display against the pale blue sky. The sun was a faint, distant orb, its muted light filtering through the trees and casting dappled shadows on the ground.

As Sophia walked deeper into the forest, she marveled at the exquisite beauty of her surroundings. The world around her seemed transformed, as if she had stepped into the pages of a fairy tale or a dream. The familiar landmarks of her usual forest walks – the gnarled old oak, the burbling brook, the moss-covered boulders – were all rendered new and mysterious beneath their frosty shroud.

The silence was almost tangible, the air so still that Sophia felt as though she could reach out and touch it. The only sounds that punctuated the quiet were the occasional creak of a swaying branch and her own steady breaths, their misty plumes dissipating into the chilly air. The absence of birdsong, the rustle of leaves, and the buzz of insects created a sense of serenity that seemed to envelop her like a comforting embrace.

As she wandered along the path, Sophia allowed her thoughts to drift, her mind meandering through memories of winters past. She recalled childhood snowball fights with her siblings, laughter ringing through the air as they dashed through the snow, their cheeks flushed with cold and exertion. She remembered the quiet, peaceful moments spent watching snowflakes drift lazily past her window, each one a tiny, intricate masterpiece.

These memories led her to think of her grandmother, whose love for winter had been infectious. They had spent many a snowy day together, wrapped in warm layers and exploring the frosty wilderness hand in hand. Her grandmother had taught her the names of the various trees and plants that peeked through the snow, their branches and leaves adorned with icy crystals. Together, they had marveled at the unique shapes and patterns of the frost on the windowpanes, and shared steaming mugs of hot cocoa, warmed by the love and companionship that defined those cherished moments.

Sophia remembered her grandmother's stories, tales of magical winter wonderlands and enchanted snowy forests, where animals spoke in hushed whispers and the air was filled with the scent of pine and woodsmoke. She had been captivated by these stories, her young imagination taking flight as her grandmother painted vivid pictures with her words, each tale a cherished gift that wove itself into the fabric of Sophia's heart.

As the years passed, their winter walks had become a cherished tradition, a time for both of them to escape the chaos of the world and find solace in the peace and beauty of the snow-covered landscape. They had forged a bond that transcended time and space, their shared love of winter a golden thread that connected them, even as the inexorable march of time carried them further apart.

Sophia's footsteps carried her deeper into the woods, the hushed, peaceful world around her seeming to slow her racing thoughts and calm her soul. She found herself drawn to a small clearing, where the trees gave way to reveal a breathtaking view of the valley below. The rolling hills, dotted with the occasional farmhouse or barn, were a study in contrasts: the deep, dark green of the evergreens standing sentinel against the brilliant white of the snow.

As she stood there, Sophia felt the weight of the world slip from her shoulders, the tranquility of the scene before her seeping into her very core. She took a deep breath, savoring the crisp, clean scent of the winter air, and felt a sense of gratitude for the beauty and serenity that surrounded her.

Slowly, she began to retrace her steps, her heart full of the quiet contentment that only a solitary walk through a snow-laden forest could bring. The silence of the woods seemed to wrap around her like a warm embrace, whispering its secrets and offering solace in its stillness.

Her thoughts turned to her grandmother once more, the memories of their shared winter walks warming her heart as she made her way back to the edge of the forest. She recalled her grandmother's words, spoken with a quiet wisdom that had resonated deep within her soul: "In the heart of winter, we find the essence of life. There is beauty in the stillness, in the hushed whispers of snowflakes as they dance on the breeze, and in the quiet moments spent with those we love."

As Sophia emerged from the forest, the golden light of the setting sun bathing the snow-covered landscape in a warm, ethereal glow, she knew that she would carry the memory of this winter's day with her always. It was not only a testament to the simple, profound beauty of nature's whispers in the heart of winter, but also a tribute to the enduring bond she shared with her beloved grandmother. The love, wisdom, and cherished moments they had shared would live on in her heart, woven into the tapestry of her life like the delicate patterns of snowflakes on a frosty winter's day.

The Art of Bonsai

Daniel carefully stepped into his small, serene workshop, his haven away from the chaotic world outside. The room was filled with a soft, diffuse light that streamed in through the frosted glass windows, casting a warm glow on the meticulously arranged rows of miniature trees that lined the shelves. The air was cool and fresh, a delicate hint of the earthy scent of soil and the sharp tang of pine lingering in the atmosphere.

He began by taking a deep, slow breath, inhaling the soothing scents around him, and closed his eyes for a moment to center himself. He could feel the gentle rise and fall of his chest, the rhythm of his breathing grounding him in the present moment. As he opened his eyes and gazed at his collection of bonsai trees, Daniel felt a familiar sense of calm wash over him, his heartbeat slowing as he lost himself in the intricate beauty of these living sculptures.

The workshop walls were adorned with shelves displaying an array of bonsai trees in various stages of development, each one unique and captivating in its own way. From the youthful, vibrant saplings to the wizened, ancient specimens, the collection represented the culmination of years of dedication and skill. The soothing sound of trickling water from a small fountain in the corner of the room added to the serene atmosphere, providing a calming backdrop to Daniel's work.

Selecting a small juniper, its delicate branches reaching out like the fingers of a dancer, Daniel carefully carried it to his work table. He placed the tree on a rotating stand, ensuring that he could access every angle of the miniature creation with ease. With a sense of reverence, he picked up his shears, the cool metal handle fitting comfortably in his hand, and began the delicate process of pruning the tree.

As he worked, Daniel focused on the subtle sensations that accompanied each snip of the shears. He felt the gentle resistance of the branches, the satisfying crunch as the shears sliced through, and the soft brush of the severed foliage as it fell away from the tree. Each cut was deliberate, a measured decision that helped to shape the tree into a harmonious reflection of nature's beauty.

Taking a moment to pause and assess his progress, Daniel circled the table, observing the juniper from every angle. He carefully considered the balance and flow of the tree's form, ensuring that the proportions were pleasing to the eye and that the branches were arranged in a manner that showcased their natural grace. As he made these assessments, he allowed his fingertips to gently trace the outline of the branches, the tactile sensation helping to guide his decision-making process.

His attention shifted to the tree's trunk, its gnarled and twisted form evoking the passage of time and the resilience of life. Daniel felt a profound sense of connection with the tree, a living being that had weathered countless seasons, its growth guided by the skilled hands of its caretaker. As he bent and shaped the branches with his fingers and wire, he was mindful of the delicate balance between control and surrender, the tree's living essence shaping his actions as much as his own will.

As the hours passed, Daniel's focus remained unwavering, his thoughts quieted by the rhythmic, meditative process of tending to his bonsai. He found solace in the slow, careful work, his awareness of his own body and the living sculpture before him merging into a seamless whole. The tension in his shoulders began to dissipate, replaced by a sense of deep relaxation that spread through his muscles like a soothing balm.

He took regular breaks to stretch and breathe, his lungs filling with the cool, fragrant air of the workshop. During these moments, Daniel marveled at the intricate beauty of his creations, the miniature trees a testament to the power of patience and perseverance. His gaze lingered on each tree, appreciating the unique qualities that made it special, from the graceful curve of a branch to the vibrant hue of its foliage.

Finally, as the sun began to set, casting a warm, golden light through the workshop windows, Daniel stepped back from the juniper and admired his handiwork. The tree had been transformed, its branches now arranged in a harmonious composition that reflected the beauty of the natural world. He felt a deep sense of satisfaction, not only in the results of his work but also in the journey he had taken to achieve them.

As he cleaned his tools and returned the juniper to its place on the shelf, Daniel took a moment to reflect on the day's work. The act of tending to his bonsai trees had not only allowed him to create something beautiful, but it had also provided him with a space for quiet contemplation, a chance to connect with his own thoughts and emotions as he engaged with the living sculptures before him.

With a final, lingering look at his collection, Daniel switched off the workshop lights and stepped out into the cool evening air. The tranquility and mindfulness that he had cultivated during his time with the bonsai trees remained with him, a reminder of the power of nature and the importance of finding moments of peace and reflection in an increasingly busy world.

Autumn's Embrace

Catherine wrapped her scarf a little tighter around her neck as she stepped out of her apartment building, ready to take on the crisp autumn day. The sky was a brilliant blue, and a gentle breeze rustled the golden leaves that had fallen from the trees, creating a mesmerizing dance on the pavement.

The park was only a short walk from her home, and Catherine had always found solace in its familiar paths and open spaces. As she strolled through the park entrance, the vivid colors of autumn surrounded her. The trees were a riot of reds, oranges, and yellows, creating a warm and inviting atmosphere that seemed to embrace her as she walked.

With each step, memories of autumns past began to flood her mind. She thought back to her childhood when her parents would take her and her younger brother, Peter, to this very park to play in the fallen leaves. Catherine recalled the excitement of waking up on a Saturday morning, knowing they would be spending the day at the park. Her mother would pack a picnic lunch, complete with her famous homemade cookies, and her father would carry a large blanket that they would spread on the ground to sit on.

Upon arriving at the park, they would spend hours jumping into the massive piles of leaves they had collected, laughing and tossing leaves in the air, as their parents watched with warm smiles on their faces. Catherine could still feel the sensation of the leaves crunching beneath her as she landed in the piles, the cool air on her cheeks, and the infectious laughter of her brother.

As she walked further into the park, Catherine's thoughts turned to her teenage years, when she and her high school friends would meet up at the park after class. The group consisted of her best friends, Sarah, Alice, and Jennifer. They would sit on the benches, wrapped in their cozy scarves and hats, sipping hot cocoa from paper cups and gossiping about the latest school drama.

Catherine remembered one particular afternoon when they had all decided to play hooky and spend the day at the park instead. It had been a crisp, sunny day, perfect for exploring the park and taking photos of the vibrant foliage. They had walked the entire length of the park, taking turns with Sarah's old Polaroid camera, capturing snapshots of their carefree youth. The park had been their sanctuary, a place where they could escape the pressures of school and simply be themselves.

Catherine passed by the small pond at the center of the park, and her memories shifted to the time she and her friends had organized a surprise birthday party for Jennifer. They had managed to gather everyone at the park without Jennifer suspecting a thing. When Jennifer finally arrived, the look of surprise and joy on her face had been priceless.

The group had spent the entire day playing games, sharing stories, and enjoying the autumn sunshine. As the sun began to set, they lit the candles on the birthday cake they had brought, and everyone sang "Happy Birthday" with gusto. The memory of Jennifer's laughter as she blew out the candles was still vivid in Catherine's mind, a testament to the deep bond they all shared.

As Catherine continued her walk, she couldn't help but smile as she recalled the countless picnics, family outings, and quiet moments of reflection she had spent in the park over the years. The park had borne witness to so many of her life's milestones, and the changing seasons had been a constant backdrop to her most cherished memories.

The gentle crunch of leaves beneath her feet brought Catherine back to the present moment, and she paused to take in the beauty of the scene before her. The sun was beginning to set, casting long shadows across the park and bathing the autumn foliage in a warm, golden light. The air was filled with the earthy scent of fallen leaves and the faint, sweet aroma of burning firewood from nearby homes. The sound of children's laughter echoed through the park, blending with the gentle rustling of leaves and the distant cawing of crows returning to their nests.

Catherine decided to sit down on a nearby bench and watch as the sun dipped below the horizon, the sky transforming into a canvas of warm hues. She closed her eyes for a moment, allowing herself to bask in the sensations of the season. The coolness of the bench beneath her, the soft breeze against her face, and the symphony of autumn sounds filled her with a sense of peace and gratitude.

As the sun finally disappeared and twilight descended upon the park, Catherine reflected on how the passage of time had not diminished the magic of the park. Despite the many changes in her life, the park had remained a constant, a place where she could always find solace and escape the demands of the world. It was a reminder of the simple joys that could be found in nature and the enduring beauty of the changing seasons.

With a contented sigh, Catherine rose from the bench and began to make her way back home, her heart full of gratitude for the memories she had created in the park and the ones she would continue to create in the years to come. As she walked, the last rays of sunlight lingered on the colorful leaves, leaving a warm glow in the autumn air. It was the perfect end to a nostalgic walk, and Catherine felt enveloped in the comforting embrace of the season as she left the park, carrying the memories of autumns past and the promise of those yet to come.